CW00923878

RACHELLE HARL.

HEALING PSORIASIS

The Ultimate Guide on How to Cure Psoriasis Naturally, Discover All the Natural Treatments For Psoriasis and Psoriatic Arthritis

Descrierea CIP a Bibliotecii Naționale a României
RACHELLE HARLAN
   HEALING PSORIASIS. The Ultimate Guide on How to Cure Psoriasis Naturally, Discover All the Natural Treatments For Psoriasis and Psoriatic Arthritis / Rachelle Harlan – Bucharest: Editura My Ebook, 2021
   ISBN

RACHELLE HARLAN

HEALING PSORIASIS

The Ultimate Guide on How to Cure Psoriasis Naturally, Discover All the Natural Treatments For Psoriasis and Psoriatic Arthritis

My Ebook Publishing House
Bucharest, 2021

TABLE OF CONTENTS

INTRODUCTION

Psoriasis is a condition that is suffered by many millions of people all over the world, with various developed countries reporting incidence rates that are remarkably similar.

For instance, in the USA, the reported rate of severe psoriasis is somewhere between 2% and 3% of the population, whilst in Australia, the condition affects around 2% of the population as well.

Furthermore, it is suggested in some quarters that up to 20% of the population of the USA may have some form of psoriasis ranging from the very mild to severe, and that perhaps as many as 4.5 million people could be serious psoriasis sufferers.

On top of this, it is reported that there are 150,000 new cases of psoriasis reported every year in the USA alone, so if it is assumed that psoriasis is as prevalent in other countries as it is in the States, it clearly represents a significant problem on a global scale.

For psoriasis sufferers, there is something of a 'good news, bad news' paradox with which most of these people have undoubtedly already learned to live.

The good news is that, on the one hand, psoriasis is not a condition that is life threatening (although it has been suggested that the condition increases the risk of heart attack). Balanced against this however is the fact that psoriasis can bring a great deal of misery to both sufferers and their families, so it is not a condition that can be ignored.

Furthermore, because it can develop into something far more unpleasant and painful, psoriasis is a condition that sufferers have to treat.

As with any medical condition or complaint, there are many different ways of treating or dealing with psoriasis, some of which are dependent on pharmaceutical drugs whilst others are completely natural. And of course, it almost always follows that treating any medical condition naturally is the best way of doing things if such treatments are going to be appropriate and effective.

The purpose of this book is to examine what psoriasis is and what causes it in greater detail, before looking at the various different ways of treating the condition.

Armed with this information, you should be in a position to consider and decide whether using pharmaceutical drugs is a good idea for treating your own psoriasis condition or whether using 100% natural methods of treating your condition is a better idea.

What is psoriasis?

Psoriasis is an inflammatory skin condition which is not contagious.

There are five different types of psoriasis, of which by far the most common is plaque psoriasis which is a form that is suffered by approximately 80% of psoriasis sufferers. This particular form of psoriasis (also known as 'psoriasis vulgaris', with the latter word meaning common) usually appears as reddish patches of raised skin which are often covered in a silvery-white scale.

These skin patches, otherwise known as plaques (hence the condition name) or lesions are most commonly found on the elbows and knees, the scalp or sometimes in the lower back area of the sufferer.

Having said this, they are not restricted to these particular areas of the body and can appear anywhere on the head, torso or limbs.

The other less common types of psoriasis are:

• Guttate psoriasis which is characterized by small red spots on the skin. This particular form of psoriasis most commonly develops in children or teenagers who have a history of streptococcal infections;

• Erythrodermic psoriasis where the patient suffers widespread redness, severe itching and often pain. This is the least common type of psoriasis which is suffered by only 1% to 2% of people who have psoriasis, which is fortunate, because this particular type of psoriasis can in the most extreme cases be life- threatening. This is because in the most severe cases, large sections of skin are shed, meaning that there are areas of exposed, unprotected flesh which could be prone to infections (it is often compared to those who have suffered very bad burns);

• Inverse psoriasis is where the sufferer is likely to find small, smooth red lesions forming in bodily skin folds where warm, moist conditions (such as in the armpits, genital area etc) encourage smooth, non-scaly but nevertheless painful to the touch plaques and

• Pustular psoriasis which is characterized by patches of red skin at the centre of which there are likely to be white pustules. This type of psoriasis occurs in less than 5% of sufferers, and is usually seen only in adults.

Irrespective of the particular type of psoriasis that an individual is suffering from, it usually causes at least a degree discomfort which in some cases can become mild to severe pain. For psoriasis sufferers, it is a fact of their life that their skin is almost always itchy, and that it can often crack and bleed as well.

In the most severe cases, the pain suffered by someone who has psoriasis can be significant enough to prevent them handling every day tasks whilst also making settled sleep extremely difficult as well.

In medical terms, the treatment that medical professionals and other doctors would recommend for psoriasis will to a very large extent depend upon the severity of the condition being suffered by the individual seeking advice.

Some dermatologists would classify psoriasis in three different categories, being mild, moderate and severe with the definition of each of these categories depending on the percentage of the patient's body that is covered with psoriasis lesions.

By these standards, anyone who has lesions cover between 5% and 10% of their body would fall into the mild category,

10% to 20% would be moderate and anyone who has more than 20% of their body covered in psoriasis lesions would fall into the severe category.

It has already been suggested that up to 20% of the population of the USA (and by extension of the rest of the Western world) may suffer psoriasis, with the vast majority falling into the mild or even very mild category. For many of these people, their condition is nothing more than a mild annoyance with moderate skin lesions and minor itching, often on a temporary basis.

At the other end of the scale, there are some unfortunates whose condition is so severe that they develop lesions all over their body and have to be hospitalized so that the condition can be treated. For these people, their psoriasis is likely to be extremely painful and in addition, it can also be disfiguring and even potentially disabling.

And unfortunately, because psoriasis is a chronic condition, meaning that it is one that is a lifelong thing, there can be no total relief for any sufferer. Psoriasis is a condition that can apparently clear up and then return (often with a vengeance) many times throughout life, and because there is no recognized cure for the condition, this is a fact that every psoriasis sufferer has to get used to and live with.

What causes psoriasis?

As with a surprising number of medical conditions, the exact causes of psoriasis have not as yet been established beyond all doubt. But, whilst the traditional view of psoriasis was that it is a condition of the epidermis, the uppermost layer of the skin, research over the past few years has begun to indicate otherwise.

This research has indicated that far from being a condition that is only related to the epidermis, the causes of psoriasis go much deeper than this. In fact, this research indicates that psoriasis is a condition that is caused by malfunctions in the sufferer's immune system when certain immune cells are activated and subsequently become overactive.

In any individual who has a perfectly normally functioning immune system, white blood cells or T-cells produce antibodies that are designed to repel bacteria and viruses. However, it is now believed that in the case of a psoriasis sufferer, these cells begin to fight an

imaginary infection or try to heal a wound that doesn't exist by creating a surfeit of new skin cells to repel the imaginary invader or to repair the nonexistent damage.

This in turn causes the plaques or skin lesions that are endemic to plaque psoriasis to appear.

Under normal circumstances, the life cycle of the average skin cell for someone who is totally healthy is around about 28 days, but it is believed that in psoriasis sufferers, their immune system is creating far too many cells. Moreover, because these cells are being produced so quickly, they mature in as little as three to six days before moving to the surface of the skin.

Consequently, because these cells are not dying quickly enough, they build up on the surface of the skin, layer upon layer, and thus the psoriatic plaques are formed.

Because of this research, we now have what is believed to be a reasonably accurate idea of what causes psoriasis.

What we do not know however is exactly why some individuals suffer from psoriasis whereas others do not.

There are on the other hand some generally accepted factors that make some individuals more likely to suffer psoriasis than others.

Why do people get psoriasis?

Research indicates that some 30% of people who develop psoriasis have a family history of the condition, but it is also true that many parents who suffer from psoriasis will have the children who have no problems of their own. On the other hand, there will be people who develop psoriasis who have no family history of the condition, so to suggest that psoriasis is hereditary could be a little misleading.

It is however true that researchers have established that there are certain genetic combinations and/or mutations that seem to make anyone who has them predisposed to suffering from psoriasis.

At the present time, researchers believe that there are nine different genetic mutations that might play a part in making certain people predisposed to suffering from psoriasis. However, there is one particular mutation of chromosome-6 known as PSORS-1 (for psoriasis susceptibility 1) which appears likely to be the particular mutation that plays the biggest role in deciding who is likely to become a psoriasis sufferer, and who is not.

According to a study published in the American Journal of Human Genetics in 2006, research has established that the role of this particular genetic mutation was seen in more than 2700 psoriasis sufferers drawn from nearly 680 families in which one or both parents were psoriasis sufferers.

It is now generally agreed within the research and scientific community that this particular mutation causes the T-cells to behave differently, hence the connection with psoriasis.

But it is also the fact that this particular genetic mutation does not necessarily mean that an individual is certain to become a psoriasis sufferer. Indeed, the same research study which was carried out by James T. Elder, MD, PhD suggests that for every individual with the PSORS-1 gene that develops psoriasis, there will be 10 other individuals carrying exactly the same gene who do not develop the condition.

Moreover, it should also be noted that many of the same mutations that are believed to make an individual predisposed to psoriasis can also have a connection with other immune mediated conditions such as type 1 diabetes or rheumatoid arthritis as well. It therefore follows that whilst some people who have a particular genetic mutation might be more prone to

16

psoriasis, it is possible that instead of psoriasis, they may suffer from diabetes or rheumatoid arthritis.

In fact, whilst the risk of developing psoriasis is increased if one or both parents are also suffererlets, the risks of developing other immune mediated conditions especially Crohn's disease or diabetes are both increased in the same situation.

From all this, it might be natural to assume that having some family history of psoriasis is likely to mean that you will develop psoriasis yourself, but in many cases, this simply does not happen.

We should therefore ask the question, why does this happen (or indeed not happen)?

Why do some people suffer and not others?

Given that there are some people whose genetic makeup makes them predisposed to suffering from psoriasis, why is it that not everyone with this particular genetic makeup suffers? Alternatively, why is it that some people with exactly the same 'psoriasis friendly' genetic makeup end up suffering from type 1 diabetes as opposed to psoriasis?

The answer seems to be that there has to be some kind of trigger to make a psoriasis sufferer's immune system start to create skin cells at such an accelerated rate that they suffer an outbreak of skin lesions.

Many different forms of triggers have been reported and suggested, such as:

- Skin abrasions, cuts and other injuries;
- Emotional stress or heightened anxiety;
- Cold, damp or cloudy weather;

- Streptococcal or other infections, including something as basic and as simple as a sore throat;

- Sunburn.

In addition, it is also believed that certain medications can bring on psoriasis as well, particularly in those who are already genetically predisposed to the condition.

Into this category fall a wide variety of drugs and medications ranging from common or garden, every day home remedies such as aspirin to beta-blockers (drugs that are used to combat high blood pressure and certain heart conditions), anti-malarial drugs and lithium.

Dermatologists have reported seeing psoriasis suddenly develop in people who have not previously had any kind of skin problems or lesions within a very short period of time after starting to take one of these medications or after they have (for example) had a sore throat or suffered sunburn.

In essence, whilst it definitely appears that those people who already have a genetic predisposition to psoriasis are more likely to develop the condition than others who do not, every individual appears to be different.

Whilst almost all psoriasis sufferers saw their condition begin because of some kind of trigger, not everyone falls into the same category.

For a relatively small number of people, psoriasis almost seems to appear out of nowhere, probably because there was some trigger in their life (for example, a relatively minor but nevertheless stressful event at the time) that they have long since forgotten.

What triggers psoriasis varies and differs from one individual to the next. Moreover, even a combination of PSORS-1 and a trigger or even several triggers does not necessarily mean that psoriasis is the inevitable result.

When does psoriasis first develop, and will I have it all my life?

As a general observation, psoriasis first develops in relatively young people, often in the teens or early adulthood. However, it is not unknown for psoriasis to be seen in children much younger than this, nor is it impossible that it can develop later in life either.

And as previously suggested, because psoriasis is a chronic condition, it is something with which a sufferer is burdened for the rest of their life.

However, this does not for a moment mean that psoriasis is a constant. Indeed, for most sufferers, it is a condition that will vary in severity throughout their life depending upon lifestyle factors at any given time.

For example, it is extremely common for someone who has psoriasis to suffer the most serious outbreaks at the times of greatest stress, whereas the opposite is also true, so that their visible psoriasis almost disappears at those times when they are at their most relaxed.

The same would also be true when you suffer an infection which can trigger an attack, whereas at times when infections are not a problem, the severity of your psoriasis is likely to recede.

When you understand the connection between your immune system and the prevalence of psoriasis, this notion of being 'attacked' when you are at your lowest makes perfectly good sense.

At such a time, your immune system is either at its weakest – when you are anxious or stressed – or alternatively at its strongest, working overtime to produce T-cells to fight infections or to heal wounds. In both cases, the crucial factor is that your immune system is imbalanced and therefore your T-cell count is also out of kilter, hence the vulnerability to an outbreak of more severe lesions.

Psoriasis and quality of your life

As highlighted previously, there are five different types of psoriasis all of which range in severity from mild to severe. However, irrespective of which particular type of psoriasis you suffer from or the degree of severity, it is a fact that any or every psoriasis sufferer can find the quality of their life is adversely affected by their condition.

For many people, even those who suffer from very mild psoriasis, anxiety, stress, loneliness, low self-esteem and a lack of confidence are constant factors in their everyday life. As there is little difference between the prevalence in psoriasis in males and females, it is very easy for sufferers of both genders to feel that their condition makes them unattractive and unpopular.

Given that most sufferers develop psoriasis in their teens and early 20s, it is particularly cruel that the condition tends to develop at a time when most people want to be at their most attractive as far as the opposite sex is concerned. Consequently, although it is entirely possible that the condition will not be physically harmful in any way, it is perfectly feasible that it could be extremely damaging in a psychological way.

This contention is borne out by one study that suggested that thoughts of suicide are three times more common in psoriasis sufferers than they were in a directly comparable control peer group of non-sufferers.

Another extremely common emotional reaction that most psoriasis sufferers will recognize is embarrassment. To put it bluntly, it is simply not nice if you recognize that you have flaky skin and that other people are made to feel uncomfortable or even repelled by your condition.

As an example, many psoriasis sufferers also suffer from scalp psoriasis, meaning that most other people probably assume that you have extraordinarily bad dandruff. This is bad enough in everyday life, but it gets considerably worse if it becomes necessary to go to the hairstylist or barber.

And, whilst psoriasis is not contagious and it is therefore not possible for anyone else to 'catch' psoriasis from a sufferer, the rest of the non- psoriasis suffering world is not necessarily always aware of this fact.

Consequently, most psoriasis sufferers report situations where other people seemed hesitant about shaking their hand or making skin to skin contact in some other way.

In addition, studies have indicated that people who suffer from psoriasis often find that life becomes increasingly frustrating as a result of their condition. This is because psoriasis often limits their ability to do the things that they did previously before the condition set in, sometimes making it difficult or even impossible to perform the basic tasks that are required as part of their normal working routine.

As a result of this, the National Psoriasis Foundation has reported that up to 56 million working hours are lost every year by psoriasis sufferers as a result of their condition. Furthermore, the same organization reported that more than a quarter of psoriasis sufferers had found it necessary to discontinue or change their normal routine daily activities as a result of psoriasis in a study carried out in 2002.

On top of all these psychological and emotional factors, there are of course many physical downsides to having psoriasis.

Itching to a greater or lesser degree is common for almost all people who have psoriasis, with cracked and bleeding skin being extremely common as well. For many people with psoriasis, pain is an everyday constant and some aspects of having the condition such as nail psoriasis can be very painful indeed.

DIAGNOSIS AND MEDICAL TREATMENTS
FOR PSORIASIS

As stated previously, there is currently no recognized cure for psoriasis.

However, there are many different forms of treatment that will be more or less effective depending upon the specific type of psoriasis that you suffer from, and the severity of your condition. Hence, there is not any one form of treatment that is used or recommended as a 'catch all' medical treatment for psoriasis.

Now, before moving to the treatment stage, the first thing that you need to do is establish that the skin complaint that you have is indeed one form of psoriasis or another. This is not possible to do on your own, so you will need to consult a dermatologist or other recognized medical practitioner for a professional diagnosis of your condition.

Once the condition that you have as been confirmed as psoriasis, it is likely that the dermatologist will recommend a particular type of treatment, the selection which depend upon a number of factors such as:

- The specific type of psoriasis that you have been diagnosed with;

- The severity of the condition, often measured by the percentage of skin affected;

- Your age, medical history and general state of health;

- The location of the psoriatic lesions and

- The overall effects that your condition appears to be having on you in terms of your physical and emotional well-being.

Once the answers to all of these questions have been established, your dermatologist is in a position to recommend a particular type of treatment for you. And again, these methods of treatment can be broken down into several different categories:

- If your psoriasis is mild to moderate, you may be recommended topical treatments, creams or lotions that can be applied to the affected area;

- Systematic treatments, those that you ingest orally or are injected might be the recommended choice is your psoriasis is more serious or

- In some cases, phototherapy (i.e. treatment by the application of light to affected areas) or laser therapy might be recommended.

Let us consider each of these different types of treatment to consider how they work, how effective they might be and whether there are any potential hazards or side-effects of which you might need to be aware.

Topical psoriasis treatments

There are various different types of topical psoriasis treatments, some of which are potentially more hazardous than others. The main treatments which are likely to come across or be recommended to buy your dermatologist or other medical practitioner are as follows.

Anthralin: Anthralin is a synthetic substitute for a naturally occurring substance known as chrysarobin which was originally extracted from the bark of the araroba tree that is most common found in South America.

The original natural substance was used as a treatment of psoriasis for at least 100 years, with both the original substance and the synthetic substitute being proved to be very effective for treating the plaques that are commonly associated with psoriasis vulgaris.

It is believed that anthralin works on psoriatic lesions by normalizing the growth rate of the skin cells, thereby gradually reducing the buildup of individual plaque areas to minimize inflammation.

Whilst anthralin is not as effective as topical steroids, it does not have the known long-term side-effects either. However, it can cause skin irritation, and it is not unknown for anthralin to leave permanent stains on almost everything it touches, including clothing and even bathroom furniture.

Coal Tar cream or ointment: As the name most probably suggests, coal tar is a thick brown liquid that is extracted as a byproduct of the carbonization of coal. It is a product that has a strong smell that many people find unpleasant or off-putting, but it is also one of the oldest known treatments for psoriasis, and in many situations, it is very effective for dealing with moderate to mild psoriasis.

There are many different coal tar psoriasis preparations, some of which can be bought over the counter at your local pharmacy or drugstore.

These different formulations are used to treat inflammation, scaling and itching, and they can come in creams that are directly applied to the affected area, shampoo (coal tar is effective for scalp psoriasis) and even in a solution that you add to your bath water which apparently helps to slow down the development of new lesions.

The main advantage of coal tar as a psoriasis treatment is that because the base materials are cheap and plentiful, the treatment itself is usually not expensive. On the other hand, many people find the smell of coal tar repugnant, and because of the dark coloration, it does have a tendency to stain everything it touches.

In addition, some psoriasis sufferers find that using coal tar over a sustained period of time can cause unpleasant skin irritation, which is a last thing anyone who has a condition which is naturally itchy needs.

Tazarotene: Tazarotene is a man-made derivative of vitamin A. that is commonly prescribed for various different types of skin afflictions, including psoriasis, sunburn and acne. It is generally used to treat mild to moderate psoriasis vulgaris, whilst it has also been used to treat nail psoriasis with a degree of success as well.

Tazarotene commonly causes local skin irritation when applied, and is known to be more effective when used in conjunction with topical corticosteroids.

It works by normalizing skin cell production activity, and is known to be effective on harder to treat areas of the body, such as knees and elbows.

However, in addition to the known skin irritation, it is known that other similar manmade derivatives of vitamin A. have been implicated in causing birth defects when taken systematically. Whilst applying such a substance topically is far less dangerous than ingesting it systematically, it is nevertheless true that using Tazarotene whilst pregnant might not be too wise.

Corticosteroids: Undoubtedly the most powerful and effective of the topical treatments for psoriasis are applied corticosteroids, but they are also the treatment that carries the greatest risk of long-term adverse side effects as well. Nevertheless, because of their effectiveness for reducing inflammation and itching whilst retarding the over-rapid rate of skin cell growth, corticosteroids are probably the most commonly prescribed topical psoriasis treatment.

Corticosteroid treatments come in various different strengths ranging from relatively mild to extremely strong, but prolonged use of these substances could have noticeable adverse side-effects. For example, it is acknowledged that corticosteroids cause thinning of the skin, excess body hair, dilate the blood vessels and they can lead to infections invading the body as well (often because of the thinned skin).

Furthermore, it is believed that they may inhibit growth in children and that long-term use renders them increasingly ineffective whilst not preventing the adverse side-effects.

The bottom line is, using corticosteroid creams, potions or lotions to treat psoriasis could result in far more problems than they solve, and it is therefore something that you want to avoid doing if at all possible.

Systematic psoriasis treatments

For moderate to milder cases of psoriasis, topical treatments are generally the first solution that a dermatologist or medical practitioner will recommend. However, in a situation where the condition is considered more serious, it is probably more likely that they will recommend some form of systematic treatment.

Given that systematic treatments are usually prescribed only for serious and severe psoriasis, it follows that the drugs being used are considerably stronger. Consequently, the potential side-effects are also far more hazardous.

Acitretin: Acitretin is a powerful vitamin A. derivative (a retinoid) that is taken orally under medical supervision. This particular systematic treatment has been shown to be effective in dealing with both erythrodermic and pustular psoriasis and works particularly well when used in combination with phototherapy.

However, the side-effects could eventually be very unpleasant or dangerous, and therefore constant medical attention and supervision is absolutely necessary. Possible side-effects include severe headaches, raised lipid levels in the blood, hair loss, dry or sticky skin and aching joints.

Cyclosporine: Cyclosporine is a very powerful immunosuppressive drug that is effective for treating severe plaque psoriasis and nail psoriasis. Whilst it is are very powerful and effective treatment, it is generally reserved for those patients for whom other forms of psoriasis treatment have not worked, owing to the possibility of severe adverse side-effects, including irreparable kidney damage.

Methotrexate: Methotrexate was one of the first commonly used chemotherapy drugs which is still used to treat moderate to severe psoriasis. Whilst it is extremely effective in doing so, it is another systematic treatment that has to be very carefully monitored because of the possibility of serious and long lasting damage to the liver.

As you will probably have gathered by now, all of the systematic psoriasis treatments that are commonly used for dealing with moderate toare are serious or severe psoriasis are extremely powerful drugs.

Consequently, it should come as no great surprise that they all have potentially serious side effects and can only be used under strict medical supervision.

Given the obvious danger inherent in taking systematic psoriasis treatments such as these, it obviously makes sense to seek natural alternatives wherever possible.

Phototherapy and laser treatment for psoriasis

Some of the treatments that have already been mentioned (e.g. acetritin) work even more effectively when they are combined with phototherapy, which is usually the application of ultraviolet light or the use of a laser.

In terms of using ultraviolet light to treat psoriasis, it is possible to undergo treatment from either ultraviolet light A or ultraviolet light B, and whilst both work in a broadly similar way, there are some differences.

In both cases, ultraviolet light is applied to the lesion area for a period of time, and in both cases, the treatment is highly effective. However, on the downside, both forms of UV treatment require many visits to the clinic or hospital over a period of time, and they do have downside as well.

In the case of UVA treatment, there is an increased risk of skin freckling, ageing and even skin cancer in a case where a patient has suffered long-term exposure to UVA light. In addition, side-effects can include nausea, headaches, burning or itching skin, irregular skin pigmentation and general fatigue.

Where UVB treatment is concerned, it is more likely that the patient will have to undergo further bouts of treatment because although the phototherapy is effectively for removing lesions, it tends to do so less permanently. And, once again, long-term exposure to UVB light increases the risk of skin cancer.

Laser therapy on the other hand is far more powerful than either of the ultraviolet light treatments, but at the same time, it is far more targeted as well. This is an advantage in one way in that using laser light to reduce or remove lesions is extremely effective, but it also means that only a relatively small area of the body can be treated at any one time.

In addition, the treatment can sometimes be painful whilst it can also cause irregular darkening of the skin and scarring as well.

Once again therefore, whilst phototherapy and laser treatment are very effective, they both have significant downsides. Consequently, you should consider the natural solutions that I'm going to propose over the next couple of chapters before subjecting yourself to potentially harmful pharmaceutical drugs or treatments that might cause complications.

However, you must also understand that there may be situations where your psoriasis is not treatable using entirely natural methods, primarily because natural treatments are almost always far gentler and less invasive than the strongest of chemical–based pharmaceuticals.

Nevertheless, unless your psoriasis is graded as serious or severe, it still makes sense to consider using natural forms of treatment before considering using powerful chemicals on or in your body.

It should only be after experimenting with natural solutions and finding that they can do nothing for you that you should resort to the chemical - based drugs that your medical attendant or dermatologist will undoubtedly recommend to you.

NATURAL TREATMENTS FOR PSORIASIS

As medical science has not yet managed to find a cure for psoriasis, it should be obvious that nature has unfortunately not to been able to provide a complete cure either.

However, there are many different natural treatments that you can try which have proved to be effective for different people at different times in alleviating, reducing or removing the plaques and lesions that are the most common external indication of psoriasis.

Unfortunately, it is almost impossible to know exactly what is going to be effective for any particular individual so to a large extent, finding what works for you is likely to be a process of trial and error. That being said, there are plenty of options that you can try to see if they alleviate or calm your condition, so all of the following alternatives are worthy of consideration.

Acupuncture for psoriasis

With its grounding in the medical practices of ancient China, acupuncture is a system of dealing with pain and treating illnesses by the application of needles to certain parts of the body. However, these needles are usually not inserted into the body at the point where the complaint or problem is most apparent, because the thinking behind acupuncture is that the body contains a network of 'highways' along which signals travel.

Consequently, it is most common for acupuncture needles to be inserted into the 'highway' at a point in the body far distant from the site of the complaint as a way of diverting signals to the places where they are supposed to go, or taking them away from the places where they are not.

However, whilst acupuncture has been used for many centuries to deal with a wide range of medical complaints and conditions, it has never been recognized as a treatment for psoriasis in China, primarily because in most Asian countries, psoriasis is a extremely rare (it is on the other hand most common in Scandinavia).

Nevertheless, Western acupuncture practitioners believe that acupuncture can be a very effective treatment for psoriasis, although there is little clinical evidence to support these assertions and what is effective in treating one person's psoriasis will vary wildly from what works best for someone else.

Although it might take a few acupuncture sessions before you see any positive, visible results the 'upside' of treating a condition with acupuncture is that there no possible side-effects. Furthermore, even if you have a fear of needles, there are many acupuncturists who now use the application of electric currents using probes rather than needles who are likely to be every bit as effective as the traditional needle brandishing acupuncturist!

You truly are what you eat!

Whilst the headline might be something of a cliché, it is never less entirely true that each and every human being on the face of the planet is made up of everything that they have ever eaten or drunk in their life. It therefore follows that in the same way as your psoriasis is a part and parcel of you, so is your diet. It is therefore not ubreasonable to assume that one has some effect on the other.

Trying to consume a diet that is going to help to keep your psoriasis under control is all about maintaining a well-balanced diet that is going to support your general well-being, whilst avoiding foodstuffs that could possibly exacerbate your situation.

For example, according to leading dermatologist Janet Prystowsky, there are many studies that support the idea that psoriasis has a tendency to cause certain nutritional deficiencies in sufferers.

Consequently, anyone who suffers from psoriasis should focus attention on replacing these missing nutrients by adding additional proteins and folates (from leafy green vegetables) to their diet. Moreover, taking on board more water and iron will not necessarily help to banish psoriasis but it will improve your well-being overall which is important, because the stronger you are, the less likely it is that you're going to suffer outbreaks of psoriatic lesions.

Whilst this will probably be no surprise, many studies have indicated that a balanced, low-fat diet can help prevent many serious medical conditions such as strokes, heart disease and cancer. What is perhaps less well-known is that some doctors have noted that the skin of psoriasis sufferers often improves when they on a well controlled weight-loss diet, whereas sufferers who are putting on additional weight are likely to see an increase in outbreaks of psoriasis.

Again, there is plenty of good sense in this, because we have already established that stress and anxiety are likely to increase outbreaks of psoriasis, whereas the opposite is also true. Working on the assumption that someone who is on a well controlled weight-loss diet is losing weight voluntarily, it naturally follows that they are happier as they are shedding the pounds, which could have some bearing on their improved condition.

The National Psoriasis Foundation suggests that they have had many reports from members that removing or at least reducing certain foodstuffs in their diet has led to significant skin improvements. Amongst the foods or ingredients listed that you should avoid are caffeine, alcohol, white flour, purified sugar and all products containing gluten.

Further tips for a diet that does not encourage the outbreak of psoriasis include:

- Consume only easily digestible food, and avoid overly spicy foodstuffs;

- Do not include too much salty, acidic or sour food in your diet;

Including more fruit and vegetables in your diet is good for general health, but it is believed that bitter gourd, steamed vegetables and pumpkin are particularly good for a 'psoriasis friendly' diet;

- Avoid too much animal fat and eggs;
- Include plenty of oily fish that is rich in omega-3 fatty acids, or failing this, take cod liver oil, lecithin or linseed oil supplements.

Other natural treatments for psoriasis

Oats: It is no coincidence that there are so many skincare products on the market that use oats as one of the main constituents, because oat extract has been used for many centuries as a soothing topical agent to manage and calm irritated or itchy skin. There are plenty of ways that you can use oats to take advantage of its soothing and calming qualities:

- Take 1 cup of dried oats and quarter of cup and dried milk before mixing it in two tablespoons of apricotskernel oil. Slowly grind the mixture together in a food blender before putting it into a muslin bag or failing that, an old sock! Drop the bag or sock into a warm bath and then gently squeeze the water from the contents of the bag onto the affected areas of your skin, as this releases the beneficial ingredients from the mixture to soothe your skin.

- Look for body lotions and moisturizers that use oats or oat extract as their main active ingredient. Apply the moisturizer liberally in the morning and in the evening, focusing in particular on any affected areas of the skin.

- Make an oat compress by wrapping oats in a bag of cloth, soaking it in buttermilk and applying the compress to any affected area of your skin. This combines two materials (oats and curd) that are both believed to have healing effects, so you should expect to see results from this particular method fairly quickly.

Aloe: There are approximately 500 different species of aloe currently known, but the one that is most commonly used and best-known is aloe vera. The secretion from the leaves of this particular plant have long since been used as a treatment for burns and minor skin damage, but in 1996, a study published in the 'Tropical Medicine and International Health' journal suggested for the first time that aloe vera could also be very effective in the treatment of psoriasis.

During this study, carried out over a period of 16 weeks, it was established that using a cream containing aloe vera indicated a significant clearing of psoriasis lesions in 25 out of 30 test individuals, compared to only 2 individuals in the control group. On the other hand, it must be said that a more recent study suggests that using commercial aloe vera may not be quite as effective as suggested but given that there is no likelihood of adverse side-effects from applying aloe vera to your plaques, it is definitely something that is worth trying as a topical treatment for psoriasis and psoriatic arthritis.

An alternative or additional way of using aloe vera to help in your fight against psoriasis is to drink the juice of the plant. Whilst some proponents of aloe vera would recommend growing your own plants from which you can expect this juice, they are notoriously difficult to grow successfully, so it is probably better to buy pre-prepared juice to drink.

The benefits of doing so are widespread, with many of these benefits being directly applicable to the psoriasis or psoriatic arthritis sufferer. For example, for the arthritis sufferer, it is known that aloe vera contains 12 completely natural substances that have been shown to counteract inflammation without any adverse side effects.

Moreover, aloe vera juice contains many vital vitamins and nutrients which will contribute to your all-round well-being, plus it has the ability to help your skin regenerate and repair itself in the quickest time possible.

Apple Cider Vinegar: Again according to the National Psoriasis Foundation, many individual members report that using apple cider vinegar has led to significant improvements in their psoriasis. These members suggest that they add the vinegar to their bath, applied directly to psoriatic nails and even applied directly to the affected areas of the skin using cotton wool balls or buds.

Alternatively, you can try to attack your psoriasis and/or psoriatic arthritis internally by adding apple cider vinegar to your diet. Whilst many people would find that drinking apple cider vinegar neat is hard going – it is very sour or bitter – you can add it to warm water with honey to sweeten the potion before drinking it. Do this at least twice a day, and you are attacking your psoriasis related problem from the inside in the most effective way possible.

The effectiveness of apple cider vinegar should not be particularly surprising because vinegar has been used throughout history as a healing solution, and the medicinal benefits of apple cider vinegar have been well known for a long time.

Capsaicin: Derived from cayenne peppers, capsaicin when applied to the skin has been shown in some studies to reduce redness, minimize scaling and to get rid of itching as well. This is believed to happen because capsaicin interrupts the activity of a molecule that affects how your brain recognizes itching and pain known as substance P.

It is for this reason that many over-the-counter arthritis pain relief products contain capsaicin, and certainly in various tests with different groups of psoriasis suffering individuals, a topical application of 0.025% cream to effected skin areas definitely reduced scaling, redness and itching.

On the downside, some individuals did report a short lived burning sensation but if you are willing to risk this happening to you, then applying a very weak capsaicin solution to your lesions could bring some much sought relief.

Tea tree oil: Tea tree oil is extracted from the Melaleuca Alternifolia tree that is native to Australia, and has been used in surgery and dentistry for nearly 100 years. Tea tree oil is widely known for its antiseptic and antibacterial qualities, and has been traditionally used for headaches, toothache, colds, rheumatism, muscle pains and skin complaints.

However, it would be singularly unwise to try to treat your toothache with tea tree oil because it is toxic if ingested. Also, it has not really been established at what level or concentration of tea tree oil it is most effective, so if you do decide to use it, you should do so with a degree of caution.

Tea tree oil is not only disinfecting and soothing, it also has the ability to penetrate deep under the skin, well below the upper epidermal level. This is particularly important for a psoriasis sufferer, because it means that the antifungal, disinfecting and healing qualities of the oil go deep under the skin, helping to regulate the production of psoriatic plaques in the earliest stages.

Although it is extremely unlikely that you will come to any real harm using tea tree oil, you should desist from using it if any skin discomfort is felt.

Milk Thistle: Milk thistle has been shown to inhibits the production of T-cells, so whilst no specific tests have been done as to how to effective milk thistle will be as a treatment for psoriasis, the fact that it can halt the growth of the cells that cause it suggests that it is worth trying. You can purchase milk thistle products at the health store or pharmacy in liquid or tablet form, and there are no adverse side-effects apart from minor gastrointestinal disturbances when you first start taking the supplement.

Oregano oil: Oregano is a commonly used spice in cooking which has antibacterial and antifungal qualities which can be helpful in keeping some of the infections that might be associated with psoriasis at bay. Oregano can be safely ingested in almost any form, and many people report that taking a daily 'dose' of oregano has significantly helped to keep their psoriasis under control.

Turmeric: Turmeric is a popular ingredient of Indian curries, and whilst you can once again buy this particular spice in food supplement form, it is easier and far cheaper to mix the spice into your food (no more than one teaspoonful is necessary). Turmeric has been shown to help reduce inflammation in every part of the body, including on the skin, as well as alleviating the pain and swelling associated with arthritis.

Shark cartilage: Studies over the past few years indicate that shark cartilage extract can help to delay the formation of new blood and skin cells which are both believed to play a significant role in the development and growth of psoriatic lesions. Shark cartilage is also believed to have highly effective anti-inflammatory qualities as well.

One particular form of shark cartilage AE-941 (known by the brand name Neovastat) has shown significant promise as a treatment for psoriasis but it is still not widely approved for general usage, because the long-term effects of usage are not known, and in the short term, it has been seen to prompt nausea and vomiting.

PSORIATIC ARTHRITIS

An overview of psoriatic arthritis

A further complication that is suffered by up to 30% of people who have psoriasis is a condition known as psoriatic arthritis.

Irrespective of which particular type of psoriasis you suffer from or the degree of severity of the condition, it is still possible to develop psoriatic arthritis, which is a lifelong condition that causes pain and stiffness in the joint, accompanied by gradual deterioration.

Signs that you might be developing psoriatic arthritis are:

• Inflamed, red psoriatic skin lesions around the joint area;

• Pain and swelling in the joints that is at its worst in the morning or following a period of rest;

- Irregularities of the finger and toe nails such as nails that begin to pull away from nail beds, pitting, an orange/yellow coloration or unusual ridge patterns.

Psoriatic arthritis is most commonly seen in the joints of fingers and toes but other critical bone joints such as knees, elbows, ankles and neck may also be affected in some individuals. No matter which joints are affected, the area surrounding the joint is almost always stiff and painful and often tends to have a darker coloration. You may also notice that the affected area feels warmer to the touch than surrounding non-affected areas.

Psoriatic arthritis can vary in severity and symptoms from one individual sufferer to another. For example, whilst some people will suffer 'full blown' psoriatic arthritis day, others might only suffer mild joint stiffness.

Furthermore, despite the name of the condition, it is not only people who have psoriasis already that will develop psoriatic arthritis.

Nevertheless, around 70% of people who develop the condition will already have psoriasis. In this situation, studies indicate that in the majority of people, arthritis will set in somewhere around 10 years after they first suffer psoriasis, although there are cases reported where arthritis begins within a matter of months of the initial psoriasis diagnosis.

As a further general guideline, the majority of people who suffer psoriatic arthritis are likely to see the first signs of the condition somewhere between their 30th and 50th birthday.

As with all forms of arthritis, psoriatic arthritis can be a debilitating and crippling condition, but unfortunately, it is extremely easy to confuse the early warning signs of the condition with dozens of other possibilities. For example, it is generally acknowledged that common early warning signs include lateral elbow pain (usually known as 'tennis elbow') or a pain in your hands or feet.

Obviously, it is extremely easy to conclude that these kinds of things can happen to anyone for any reason and to simply ignore them, especially if there are no recognizable plaques visible or evident. In a similar manner, pain in the shoulder, neck or upper back could be the first signs of psoriatic arthritis, but once again, these warning signs would be extremely easy to mistake for 'just one of those things' to be ignored as a result.

However, once psoriatic arthritis begins to set in, approximately 9 out of every 10 people who suffer will begin to see the condition manifest itself through the nails of their fingers and toes. In this case, the individual concerned might start to see their nails begin to pull away from the nail bed or for pitted marks and discoloration to become evident.

As soon as any such physiological changes become evident, it is extremely important that anyone who suffers from psoriasis should consult their medical practitioner immediately, because it is possible for joint deterioration to be halted with appropriate treatment.

And of course, there are natural treatments that you can use to offset the worst effects of psoriatic arthritis, but we will return to those a little later.

Perhaps not surprisingly, psoriatic arthritis and its effects range in severity from individual to individual. However, the effects of psoriatic arthritis can be extremely severe.

For instance, according to statistics from the National Psoriasis Foundation, around one in every five people who suffer psoriatic arthritis have damage in five or more joints of their body, meaning that their quality of life and ability to complete basic, everyday tasks is severely impaired.

And then of course there are people at the opposite end of the spectrum who suffer nothing more than a slight stiffness in the joints. However, even for these people, it has to be accepted that the condition can always worsen.

What causes psoriatic arthritis?

Even in people who contract psoriatic arthritis who were not previously psoriasis sufferers, it is generally believed that the primary cause of psoriatic arthritis is remarkably similar to those of psoriasis.

For instance, it seems likely that psoriatic arthritis is caused by a defect in the sufferers immune system. Furthermore, it seems likely that those who suffer psoriatic arthritis are often genetically predisposed to do so and they need some kind of psychological, emotional or physical trigger to bring on the onset of arthritis in exactly the same way as there is with psoriasis.

Who is likely to suffer from psoriatic arthritis?

In the USA, there are believed to be around one million people who suffer from psoriatic arthritis, with the majority of those people having previously been psoriasis sufferers, particularly sufferers from pustular psoriasis.

Most commonly, the effect of psoriatic arthritis will be felt by people who are already psoriasis sufferers who are between the age of 30 and 50. However, it is not unknown for even young children to develop psoriatic arthritis.

Girls from as young as 2 to 4 years of age have been known to suffer psoriatic arthritis, with the prime time for the condition to take hold in children being around 11 or 12 years of age for both boys and girls.

Most worryingly, it is even known for arthritis to set in even before psoriasis has appeared, although because it is extremely rare, this would not necessarily be something that most parents with no family background of psoriasis should be overly concerned about.

Diagnosis and recognizing the symptoms of psoriatic arthritis

The number one goal for anyone who suspects that they might be susceptible to psoriatic arthritis is to know how to recognize the onset of the condition as early as possible.

Of course, the condition is not called psoriatic arthritis for nothing. The majority of people who suffer are those who have previously suffered psoriasis, so that would be the first clue that you might these susceptible to the condition.

Secondly, any unexplained aches or pains particularly around the joints might be giving you a clue that psoriatic arthritis is 'targeting' you. The majority of sufferers are within a certain age band (30-50), so is this where you are?

It is important to understand that once psoriatic arthritis sets in, joint deterioration and the corresponding increase in pain can begin to accelerate very quickly, so you must do something to put the brakes on this acceleration.

As most people who have ever encountered someone who is suffering from arthritis probably understand, it is not a particularly difficult condition to recognize, but it is not easy to recognize the difference between different types of arthritis if you're not medically qualified.

After all, how many non-qualified individuals would be able to differentiate between someone suffering from rheumatoid arthritis or psoriatic arthritis?

The bottom line is, if you do nothing about psoriatic arthritis, it is perfectly feasible that you're going to end up being able to do nothing about anything owing to your condition. It is therefore imperative that if you have any reason to suspect that you might have a problem, you consult a dermatologist or other recognized medical professional as quickly as possible.

MEDICAL TREATMENT
FOR PSORIATIC ARTHRITIS

The goals of treating psoriatic arthritis can be broken down into three different categories. These are:

- To first control the symptoms;
- Next to inhibit and control joint damage and deformities and finally
- To prevent disability.

However, every single psoriatic arthritis sufferer is different, and therefore no single medical treatment will solve everyone's problems. For this reason, there are many different specific formulations of different drugs used to treat psoriatic arthritis sufferers, but the majority of these drugs fall under one of two categories.

Consequently, rather than dealing with every individual drug, it makes more sense to look at the two different classes of drug to explain why they work and the potential adverse side-effects of each.

Nonsteroidal anti-inflammatory drugs (NSAIDs): NSAIDs are drugs that help to alleviate pain, ease the stiffness in joints and take down swelling that is all too commonly associated with every form of arthritis. These particular drugs are very commonly used by non- psoriatic arthritis sufferers, and can include such common household medicines as aspirin and ibuprofen.

Obviously, the potential side-effects of the particular NSAID that you are taking will vary from one medicine to another, but they can include nausea, headaches, vomiting, diarrhea, suppressed appetite and dizziness. They can also encourage water retention which in turn might encourage edema, and in a worst-case scenario, they can cause kidney or liver failure, ulcers and prolonged internal bleeding, particularly after surgery.

Disease-Modifying Anti-Rheumatic drugs (DMARDs): Using DMARDs is generally considered to represent a less effective way of treating psoriatic arthritis, because whilst they slow down the development of the condition, they very rarely
60

stop or reverse it altogether. Also, because in many cases it takes the drug in question anywhere from six to eight months to have any positive effect, they are generally also considered to be slow acting drugs as well.

Although it is not fully understood how DMARDs work, it is generally agreed that they effect a slowdown in the advance of psoriatic arthritis by slowing or modifying the activities of the immune system of the sufferer in some way.

However, once again, depending upon the particular type of drug that is prescribed to you, you have to be aware that there are potential of unpleasant and dangerous side-effects.

These include stomach pain, diarrhea or constipation, nausea, vomiting, headache and possibly a violent skin rash. Then there are potentially even more dangerous side effects such as increased blood pressure, lowered white cell count (which may partly explain why they are effective in treating a psoriasis related condition), hair loss and increased susceptibility to infection.

As with psoriasis itself, you cannot fail to arrive at the conclusion that in some cases, the treatments that your dermatologist or medical attendant might recommend to you could in some cases be as bad as if not worse than the medical condition that they are prescribed to treat.

NATURAL TREATMENTS
FOR PSORIATIC ARTHRITIS

Natural chemicals and devices for the relief of psoriatic arthritis

It is perhaps not too surprising that many of the natural treatments that you might use for psoriasis can also be effective for helping to deal with the swelling, stiffness and joint pain that is associated with psoriatic arthritis as well.

For example, topically applied Tea Tree Oil is known to relieve muscle and joint pain, whereas adding turmeric to your food or taking it as a food supplement can help to relieve the inflammation and pain associated with any form of arthritis.

However, because psoriasis and psoriatic arthritis are two very different conditions, there are many other natural treatments that are worthy of your consideration if you suffer from psoriatic arthritis that may not be quite so applicable in the case of psoriasis.

Chondroitin and Glucosamine: Chondroitin and Glucosamine are both natural sulphate solutions that you can use to reduce the pain and slow the advancement of osteoarthritis, which is the deterioration of the cartilage between your bone joints. Both of these substances occur naturally in the body, with chondroitin believed to improve water retention which in turn maintains elasticity in the cartilages between the bones, whereas glucosamine promotes the repair and production of the cartilage.

The National Psoriasis Foundation suggests that there are very few side - effects with either of these substances and that their long-term safety record is already well established. However, pregnant women or those who are trying to become pregnant should not take them, and glucosamine is likely to increase blood sugar levels, so it is not advisable for diabetics.

These can both be found in tablet form at health stores, as can all of the following supplements as well.

S-Adenosyl methionine (SAM-e): SAM-e is a synthetic version of a chemical that is naturally manufactured by all animals. It helps to make and regulate hormones and neurotransmitters, which in turn regulate mood and emotions.

More importantly for a psoriatic arthritis sufferer, SAM-e is involved in the manufacture of glutathione which the liver uses as part of the process of removing toxins from the body (toxins which can exacerbate both psoriasis and psoriatic arthritis) whilst it is also instrumental in helping to rebuild cartilage which once again reduces the pain and incidence of osteoarthritis.

Methylsulfonylmethane (MSM): MSM which is sometimes known as dimethyl sulfone is a natural chemical which is found in fruits, plants and grains that is unfortunately destroyed by the body during food digestion.

In order to repair and maintain healthy joint functions and connective tissues, the body needs sulfur. Consequently, MSM is able to help the psoriatic arthritis sufferer because it is a natural sulfate which supplements the often-too low levels of sulfate that most people have. It is also reported that MSM has pain relieving qualities and the ability to reduce inflammation, but there is little established evidence of why this should be.

It should also be noted that there is little scientific data on the long - term benefits or side-effects of using MSM, so it should be used with a degree of caution.

Herbs to treat psoriatic arthritis

Nettles: Nettles are found almost everywhere, but they are nevertheless a true wonder food supplement from nature. Including nettles in your diet can help reduce high blood pressure, minimize the worst effects of eczema and relieve the pain and swelling associated with rheumatism.

Saffron: Saffron is a natural source of weak hydrochloric acid which helps to banish uric acid from the body, which is beneficial because it is uric acid that bonds the extra calcium deposited in the bone joints to the bone itself. It also helps to reduce the buildup of lactic acid as well.

Yucca extract: In testing over the past two years, it has been indicated that including yucca extract in their diet helped many arthritis sufferers to reduce the severity of their condition. Whilst you may be able to find yucca extract–based supplements in health food stores already, tests are still going on.

Nevertheless, thus far, the results seem extremely encouraging for anyone who suffers from any form of arthritis or rheumatism.

Bogbean: Bogbean is an ancient remedy that has proved to have significant anti-inflammatory and tonic qualities, something that is therefore an ideal treatment for an arthritic condition.

CONCLUSION

As highlighted throughout this book, whilst there are many chemical drug based treatments available for both psoriasis and psoriatic arthritis, there are also a wide range and number of natural treatments for both of these conditions as well.

And as with almost any medical condition, because most natural treatments have few adverse side-effects (if any), it always make sense to consider using a natural treatment method before using chemical drug-based solutions that may treat the condition but cause other problems in the process of doing so.

For anyone who suffers from psoriasis, it is an unfortunate fact that there is no known cure for the condition at present. However, as you should understand by now, there are plenty of natural treatments that you can use to deal with your psoriasis or indeed with psoriatic arthritis that can reduce or even eliminate the worst effects of the condition.

Of course, you should not totally ignore medical advice or recommendations, especially if your psoriasis or psoriatic arthritis is particularly severe. In some circumstances, there is no doubt that medical intervention is likely to be necessary in order to bring the worst cases of psoriasis and psoriatic arthritis under control and if this is the case for you, you may need to heed medical advice.

However, in many cases, drug-based pharmaceuticals that can be used topically or systematically will automatically be recommended by your medical adviser irrespective of how serious your psoriasis psoriatic arthritis is. In such circumstances, it may be that natural solutions could provide exactly the same amount of relief as pharmaceutical drugs.

Hence, once you know that psoriasis or psoriatic arthritis is your problem, it will surely make sense to try natural solutions before reverting to pharmaceuticals.

Psoriasis is a condition that can be a blight on your life, but it does not have to be. Equally as importantly, it is a condition that can be treated entirely naturally.

Armed with the information that you have read of in this book, now is the time to start dealing with psoriasis in a completely natural manner.

CPSIA information can be obtained
at www.ICGtesting.com
Printed in the USA
LVHW030705241121
704256LV00012B/1272